Low-Impact Exercise for Seniors

Your Guide to Healthy Aging Through Movement

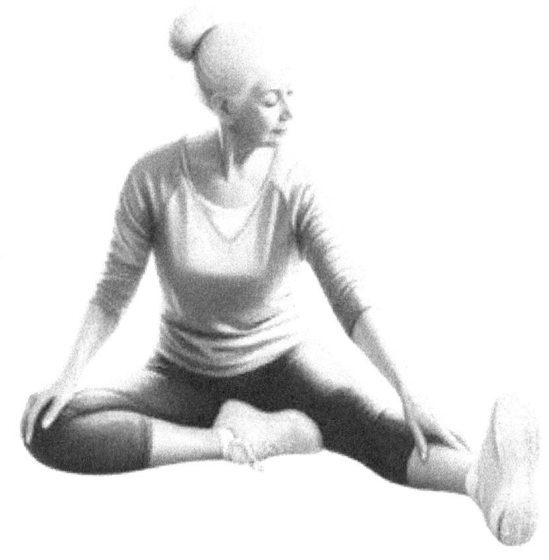

By Desmond T. Hall

Copyright © 2024 by Desmond T. Hall

Declaimer ▲

This book is a work of nonfiction. Names, characters, places, and incidents are either the product of the author's imagination or are used fictitiously. Any resemblance to actual persons, living or dead, business establishments, events, or locales is entirely coincidental.

TABLE OF CONTENT

INTRODUCTION

Remember how you felt after completing a difficult hike? Laughter erupting during a rousing game of tag with grandchildren? That vivid, young vitality coursing through your veins, buddy, does not fade with age. It's sleeping, ready to be roused by the power of low-impact exercise.

Consider this: You are not restricted to treadmills or filthy exercise bikes. Imagine yourself flowing elegantly through a tai chi exercise in the morning sun, your muscles humming with fresh strength. Feel the energizing flow of a morning stroll, the crunching of leaves under your feet, the wind whispering whispers of possibilities.

This isn't a fantasy; it's your invitation to an adventure park designed exclusively for experienced adventurers like you. Low Impact Exercise for Seniors is your map, compass, and guide to rediscovering the delight of movement and the gleeful defiance of time's restrictions.

Forget about aching bones and creaking joints. We're here to portray a future in which stairs become springboards and balancing is an elegant dance rather than a struggle. We'll provide you with mild, efficient workouts that will shape your body, improve your intellect, and energize your soul without any hardship.

This isn't a book about constraints; it's a transformational toolset. We have a path for you regardless of your fitness level, whether you haven't exercised in years or want to push yourself beyond your present routine.

So, are you ready to ditch your rocking rocker in favor of a bright tapestry of motion? Let's turn the page, enter the theme park, and rewrite the story of aging together.

Dive into the first chapter to reawaken your inner adventurer. Your body, mind, and spirit are all anticipating this journey.

OTHER BOOKS BY THIS AUTHOR

Scan the QR Code Below to Get Access

CHAPTER 1

The Importance of Low-Impact Exercise for Seniors

Our bodies murmur changes as we elegantly tread the road of time. Joints creak a little, strength fades, and the brilliant vitality of youth fades into the distance. Instead of surrendering to the perceived constraints of aging, there is a potent antidote: low-impact exercise.

It's a common fallacy that physical exercise grows increasingly harmful with each passing year. In reality, low-impact exercise for seniors is not only helpful, but also necessary. It's a bright tapestry woven with strands of better health, lifted spirits, and a revitalized sense of self-sufficiency.

Imagine this:

- Stronger, more stable you: Tai chi and water aerobics gently shape muscles, enhance balance, and lessen the chance of falling, keeping you securely planted in life's adventures.
- A joyfully dancing heart: Gentle activity gets your blood moving, fueling your heart, brain, and all of your cells. It's a natural elixir of vitality that improves cognitive function and lowers the risk of chronic illnesses.
- Pain fades, replaced by sunshine: Low-impact exercises reduce joint tension, relieving aches and pains and allowing you to fully participate in the activities you like.
- A mind in full bloom: Physical activity is a powerful antidepressant, reducing stress and anxiety while improving mood and sharpening attention. It's like a spa for your spirit, promoting calm and well-being.
- Independence with a glimmer: Strong muscles and greater stamina allow you to easily do routine duties.

Climbing stairs, carrying groceries, and even gardening become delightful manifestations of your own competence.

Low-impact exercise does not include strenuous workouts or exceeding one's physical limits. It's a movement festival, a rediscovering of the inherent delight in stretching, swaying, and feeling your body come alive. It's about carving out time for yourself, time to connect with your breath, your power, and the simple thrill of movement.

It is about reinventing the story of age. It's all about swapping out the rocking chair for a springboard and exchanging creaking joints for a symphony of muscle. It's about choosing to embrace time's knowledge while delighting in your spirit's vitality.

So, dear friend, come out of the shadows and into the light of motion. There's an adventure park waiting for you, one that's lined with moderate activities and brimming with life's bright energy. Take a deep breath, turn the first page, and enjoy the ride. Your body, mind, and soul are all ready to soar.

Remember that age is only a number. Your capacity for living a healthy, pleasant life is limitless. Allow low-impact exercise to be your guide and partner on this exciting journey of rediscovery.

Begin moving, flourishing, and enjoying your most energetic life ever.

Health Benefits of Low-Impact Exercises

The human body is a beautiful mechanism built for motion. However, as we age, that perfectly tuned engine begs for changes. Once our allies, high-impact exercises might now seem jarring, leaving us achy and disheartened.

However, this does not imply that movement has become a distant memory. Enter the realm of low-impact exercise, a soothing symphony of health benefits that will leave you feeling energized rather than frustrated.

1. A Dancing Heart: Our hearts enjoy the gentle push of low-impact exercises since they are constantly pumping lifeblood. Walking, swimming, and yoga all increase blood flow, which lowers your risk of heart disease, stroke, and high blood pressure. It's like a natural tune-up, keeping your cardiovascular system humming with energetic rhythm.
2. Muscle Melody: While age may cause muscle atrophy, low-impact training provides a harmonizing contrast. Pilates and tai chi gently shape and build, increasing balance, reducing falls, and making daily activities easier. Consider facing stairs with increased ease, with the assurance of a body that says, "Yes!" to your experiences.
3. Bone Harmony: The brittle dance of weakening bones, osteoporosis, throws a shadow on aging. Low-impact workouts, such as weight training and dance, provide an effective counter-balance. They promote bone development, improving density and resilience while keeping you securely rooted in the present. Consider it like writing a symphony of strong bones, a tune that resonates with independence and confidence.
4. Joint Jubilation: Aching joints can make mobility a painful challenge. Low-impact exercise, on the other hand, is a calming salve. Water aerobics and elliptical exercise reduce joint stress, lowering discomfort and inflammation. It's a lullaby for your joints, urging them to join the happy chorus of pain-free mobility.
5. Mindful Movement, Mood Magic: The mind and body are constantly tangoing, and low-impact exercise enters the beat beautifully.

Yoga and meditation lower stress and anxiety while improving mood and cognitive performance. It's like a spa day for your spirit, washing away negativity and leaving you calm, focused, and ready to embrace the possibilities of life.

6. Independence Encore: Low-impact exercise is a celebration of freedom as well as physical rewards. With stronger muscles and better balance, everyday chores become a beautiful dance rather than a frustrated battle. Carrying groceries, caring to the garden, and even visiting new locations become testaments to your newly discovered independence.

7. Diabetes Control: Chronic Disease Management Regular physical activity helps maintain blood sugar levels, thus low-impact workouts are excellent for diabetics.

8. Arthritis Relief: The mild nature of low-impact activities relieves arthritis symptoms by increasing joint mobility and decreasing inflammation.

9. Stability and Balance: Improved Stability: Low-impact workouts that focus on balance and coordination help to enhance stability, lowering the risk of falling. This is especially important for elders, who may be more vulnerable to balance-related mishaps.

So, why settle for a life limited by constraints? Low-impact exercise encourages you to turn up the volume on your health, strength, and joy. It's a prelude to a dynamic encore, in which your body transforms into a powerful and graceful instrument, playing the lovely music of a life well-lived. Don't allow your inner dancer be silenced by your age. Pick up the beat of low-impact exercise and let the song of your health and pleasure to fill the air.

Mental Well-being and Exercise

The complicated dance between mental health and exercise produces a dynamic relationship, with each profoundly impacting and uplifting the other. Understanding how physical activity contributes to emotional and psychological well-being is becoming increasingly important as the world realizes the importance of mental health. This body-mind synergy is more than simply endorphins; it's a comprehensive strategy to building resilience, battling stress, and cultivating a happy outlook.

Imagine this scenario: you lace up your shoes, head out into the cool morning air, and go for a quick walk. A small change happens when your legs pump and your lungs fill with oxygen. Stress begins to fade, and a serene calm replaces it. Worries, which were once menacing giants, have shrunk into manageable pebbles. This, my friend, is the mind-altering power of exercise.

- Stress Slayer: The modern world bombards us with stresses, and our thoughts may short-circuit like overloaded circuits. Exercise is an excellent circuit breaker. Endorphins, our bodies' natural feel-good chemicals, are released during physical exertion. These endorphins counteract stress chemicals, leaving you feeling calmer, more focused, and ready to tackle the difficulties of the day.
- Anxiety Remedy: Anxiety's crushing grasp may make us feel confined, our minds racing with unpleasant ideas. Exercise provides a means of escape. You may break away from mental chatter by focusing on the movement of your body and the rhythm of your breath. Exercise also increases self-efficacy, or belief in one's capacity to cope, giving you the courage to face your fears one step at a time.

- Mood Maestro: Are you feeling down? Exercise can serve as your own mood controller. Physical exercise increases the synthesis of neurotransmitters such as serotonin and dopamine, which are important for mood regulation and reducing depression symptoms. Consider it like tuning your mental symphony, harmonizing your emotions into a joyous tune of well-being.
- Memory Loss: Cognitive Cadence? Is your mind foggy? Exercise can help you to sharpen your mental edge. Physical activity improves cognitive function and memory by increasing blood flow to the brain. It also encourages the development of new brain cells, which keeps your mental engine functioning smoothly and effectively.
- Confidence Conductor: Exercise is about shifting your self-perception as well as your physique. As your strength and resilience improve, so will your confidence. You overcome self-doubt, enjoy your accomplishments, and embrace the bright, competent individual that you are. This increased confidence pervades all facets of your life, enabling you to face problems and pursue your objectives.

But keep in mind that no elaborate choreography is required for this mental dance. It's not about punishing exercises or pushing yourself to your limits. Find your joyful activity, whether it's a brisk walk in the woods, a peaceful yoga class, or a raucous dance party in your living room. The idea is to engage in things that make you feel alive and connected to your body.

So get your body moving and watch your intellect grow. Allow exercise to be your personal therapist, mood booster, and confidence builder. It's a voyage of self-discovery, a route to a happier, more resilient person, not simply a healthier body. Lace up your shoes, walk outside, and enjoy the magnificent symphony of mental well-being that begins to play the instant you move.

Keep in mind that your body and mind are not distinct creatures; they work in perfect unison. The conductor is exercise, who leads them both in a joyful ballet of well-being. So take responsibility, turn on the music, and see your mental health improve with each step you take.

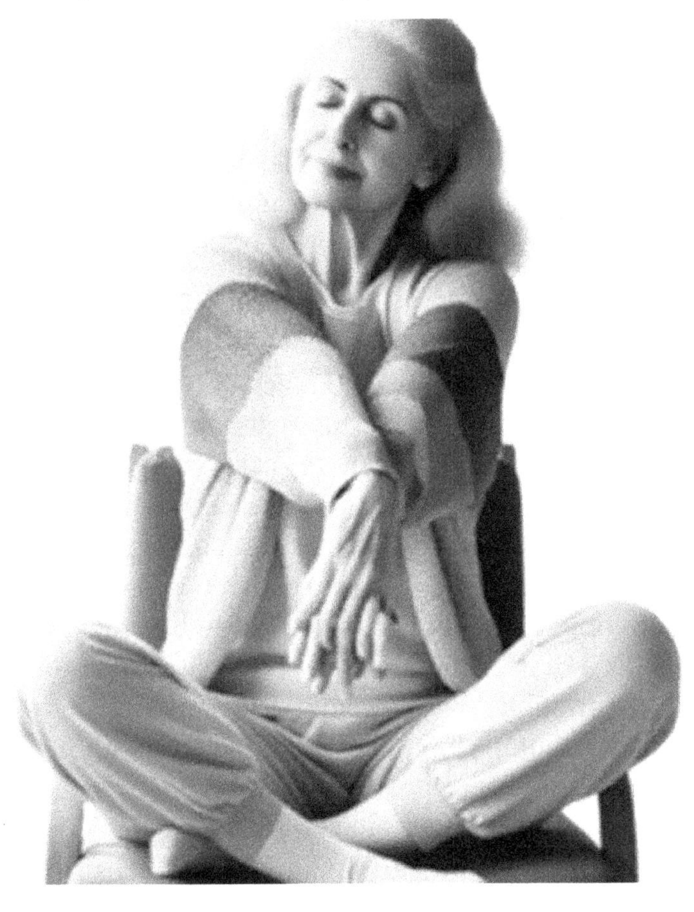

CHAPTER 2

Tailoring Exercises to Seniors' Needs

When it comes to senior exercise, one-size-fits-all is no longer an option. Each senior is as unique as a snowflake, with individual talents, limits, and fitness objectives. That's where customized workouts come in, turning your workout from a chore into a celebration of your unique requirements and goals.

Instead of straining with heavy weights or bouncing uncomfortably on a treadmill, imagine gliding through a tai chi practice, feeling your strength and balance grow. Imagine yourself dancing to upbeat music, laughing as you rediscover the joy of movement. This is the power of customized exercise for elders.

- Focus on Function, Not Fads: Forget about pursuing exercise fads aimed at younger bodies. Functional movements that mirror daily tasks should be prioritized in senior exercise. Climbing stairs, carrying groceries, and even gardening become fitness criteria, guaranteeing that workouts transfer into real-life strength and independence.
- Whisper of Wisdom, Pay Attention to Your Body: No more ignoring tiny pains or pushing through agony. Senior exercise is a dialogue with your body, an elegant dance in which restrictions are recognized and changes are welcomed. Gentle chair exercises, water workouts, and even modified yoga positions are all alternatives for making workouts pleasurable and safe.
- Muscle loss is a natural part of aging, but it doesn't have to be a death sentence for strength. Low-impact strength exercise with resistance bands, small weights, or even your own bodyweight can increase muscle mass, bone density,

and self-esteem. Consider it as a whisper to your muscles, reminding them of their inner strength.

- Balance and Movement Harmony: Falling is a common concern for seniors, but fear should not determine movement. Balance activities such as tai chi, yoga, and even standing on one leg for brief periods of time may increase stability and confidence, allowing you to stay securely planted in life's experiences.

- Mind, Body, Spirit Symphony: Senior exercise is about a comprehensive approach to well-being, not simply muscles. Yoga and meditation can help to decrease stress and anxiety, enhance cognitive function, and cultivate a sense of peace and clarity. Consider it like tuning the strings of your mind, body, and soul to create a vivid symphony of happiness.

- Finding Your Joyful Movement: Senior exercise should, above all, be a celebration, not a duty. Find hobbies that you actually like, such as dancing, swimming, strolling with friends, or gardening. When movement brings you joy, it becomes sustainable, converting your routine into a brilliant tapestry of laughter, strength, and a revitalized enthusiasm for life.

Note, that age is only a number. Your capacity for living an active, pleasant life is limitless. Allow personalized exercise to be your guide and partner on this thrilling journey of rediscovery. Move with intention and enthusiasm, and watch your life flourish with each stride you take.

Common Health Concerns Among Seniors

Our bodies murmur changes as we elegantly tread the road of time. While these whispers may occasionally become shouts, recognizing prevalent health problems among seniors equips us with information and strength to address them.

1. The Cardiovascular Chorus: Because our hearts are constantly pumping lifeblood, they might become vulnerable to cardiovascular disorders such as heart disease and stroke. High blood pressure, high cholesterol, and a lack of physical exercise might form a troubling chorus. Fortunately, a good diet, regular exercise, and stress management can help to harmonize this song and keep our hearts singing loudly.

2. The Creaky Bone Ballet: As we age, we lose sight of bone health, which can lead to osteoporosis, a condition in which bones become brittle and prone to fractures. Calcium and vitamin D, as well as weight-bearing sports like weight training and dancing, can help to counteract this fragility dance. Building strong bones allows us to confidently face life's challenges.

3. The Joint Jangle: Joint aches and pains can cause movement to seem jumbled. Conditions such as arthritis and rheumatism can make daily duties difficult. Gentle workouts such as tai chi and swimming, along with a healthy weight, can alleviate the jangle and restore harmony to our movement.

4. The Memory Maze: The mind, which was once a lively marketplace of memories, can occasionally become lost in a hazy maze. Cognitive decline and dementia might become unpleasant visitors in our mental chambers. Engaging in cognitively engaging activities such as reading, puzzles, and social interactions might help us traverse cognitive problems by lighting a candle in the maze.

5. The Emotional Ebb and Flow: Life is full of ups and downs, and seniors are especially sensitive to despair and anxiety.

These emotional floods might draw us under, but reaching out for help, practicing mindfulness, and engaging in things that bring us joy can be life rafts that keep us afloat and allow us to appreciate the sunlight.

Remember that these health issues are not unavoidable notes in the symphony of aging. We may dial down the volume on these worries and keep the music of our lives lively and happy by taking a proactive approach, embracing healthy behaviors, and getting medical guidance when necessary.

Living well in our latter years entails recognizing our body, embracing preventative actions, and honoring our inherent resilience. Allow education to be our conductor, healthy habits to be our instruments, and joy to be the melody that fills our hearts with each passing year.

Customizing Exercises for Specific Conditions

Forget about cookie-cutter workouts; tailoring activities to individual circumstances is the key to living a healthy, pain-free life. Each of us has a unique story that is intertwined with our talents, limits, and health issues. Recognizing this uniqueness is the key to unlocking the enchantment of tailored exercise, which transforms movement from a duty to a celebration of well-being.

- Consider this: instead of fighting your body's whispers, you listen closely and design activities that respect your limits while amplifying your capabilities. A sprained knee does not have to put an end to your fitness journey; instead, it serves as an encouragement to try low-impact swimming or modified yoga positions. A little arthritis in your hands is not a hindrance, but rather a prompt to try chair exercises or resistance bands adapted to your grip. This is the power of conditional customization.

- Focus on Function, Not Fads: Instead of a one-size-fits-all approach, promote functional motions that reflect your everyday life. Climbing stairs, carrying groceries, and even gardening become fitness criteria, ensuring that workouts transfer into real-world strength and independence. Imagine accomplishing routine activities with ease, a tribute to the power of individualized movement.

- The Wise Whisperer advises you to pay attention to your body: No more ignoring tiny pains or pushing through agony. Customized exercise is a dialogue with your body, an elegant dance in which limits are acknowledged and adaptations are accepted. Gentle cardio for heart ailments, modified balancing exercises for joint disorders, even water workouts for chronic pain - the possibilities are unlimited for making activities fun and safe.

- Muscle loss may be a quiet companion of age or a result of certain illnesses, but it does not have to imply weakness. Low-impact strength exercise targeted to your specific needs can help you gain muscle, enhance bone density, and raise your confidence. Consider it as a whisper to your muscles, reminding them of their underlying strength, even if certain changes are required.

- Balance, Movement Harmony: Falls can be a troubling melody for many, but fear should not govern movement. Balance activities, such as tai chi, yoga, or simple standing challenges, may increase stability and confidence, keeping you securely planted in life's adventures. Consider moving with greater elegance, evidence of the harmony attained via individualized balancing training.

- Mind, Body, Spirit Symphony: Customized exercise is about a comprehensive approach to well-being, not simply muscles. Adapted yoga and meditation can help you decrease stress and anxiety, improve cognitive function, and cultivate a sense of peace and clarity. Consider it like tuning the strings of your mind, body, and spirit to create a dynamic symphony of well-being, even when certain situations are present.

- Finding Your Joyful Movement: Personalized exercise should, above all, be a joy, not a duty. Find things that you actually like, whether it's adapted dancing, swimming with pals, or chair-based workouts that make you giggle. Movement that brings you joy becomes sustainable, converting your routine into a vivid tapestry woven with confidence, strength, and a revitalized enthusiasm for life.

Remember that your age and certain problems are only a portion of your own tale. Your capacity for living an active, pleasant life is limitless. Allow customized exercises to be your guide and friend on this exciting journey of rediscovery. Move with purpose, move with joy, and watch your life flourish in your own unique manner with each stride you take.

Consulting with Healthcare Professionals

As a senior, embarking on a low-impact fitness program is an exciting step toward vitality and independence. But, before you put on your walking shoes, keep in mind that consultation with healthcare professionals is the key to a safe and genuinely effective voyage.

Consider these professionals to be your guides and allies:

- Choosing a Personal Path: No two bodies are similar, and aging adds another element of uniqueness. Healthcare specialists can understand your health narrative, identifying strengths and weaknesses and designing an exercise regimen that is tailored to your specific requirements. There will be no cookie-cutter routines, simply a personalized road map to joyous, pain-free mobility.

- Safety First, Always Confidence: Aging, chronic diseases, and even drugs can complicate the fitness equation. Consulting with a healthcare expert ensures that your fitness path is safe and sustainable, limiting dangers while optimizing benefits. It's like having a fitness guardian angel that celebrates your victories and keeps you on track.
- Motivation is important: Let's face it, even the most ardent self-starters want encouragement. Healthcare experts may be your steadfast encouragement and guiding compass. They'll applaud your achievements, give you light nudges when required, and remind you of the tremendous progress you're making. Consider them your personal coach for your complete health journey, not just your body.
- Beyond Movement: Exercise is only one piece of the jigsaw that is well-being. Healthcare specialists may offer comprehensive advice on nutrition, sleep, stress management, and any other aspects affecting your health. It's like having a personal life coach who optimizes your entire live to create a harmonic symphony of happiness.

Consulting with healthcare specialists is a power move, not a show of weakness. It's as simple as stating "I choose to invest in my health, and I want the best possible roadmap to get there." It's about realizing the full potential of low-impact exercise, about moving into a future where movement is associated with joy, confidence, and a rich existence that's uniquely suited to you.

Remember that your health is the most valuable investment you will ever make. Seek professional advice, discover your personal path to well-being, and watch yourself blossom into the healthiest, happiest version of yourself.

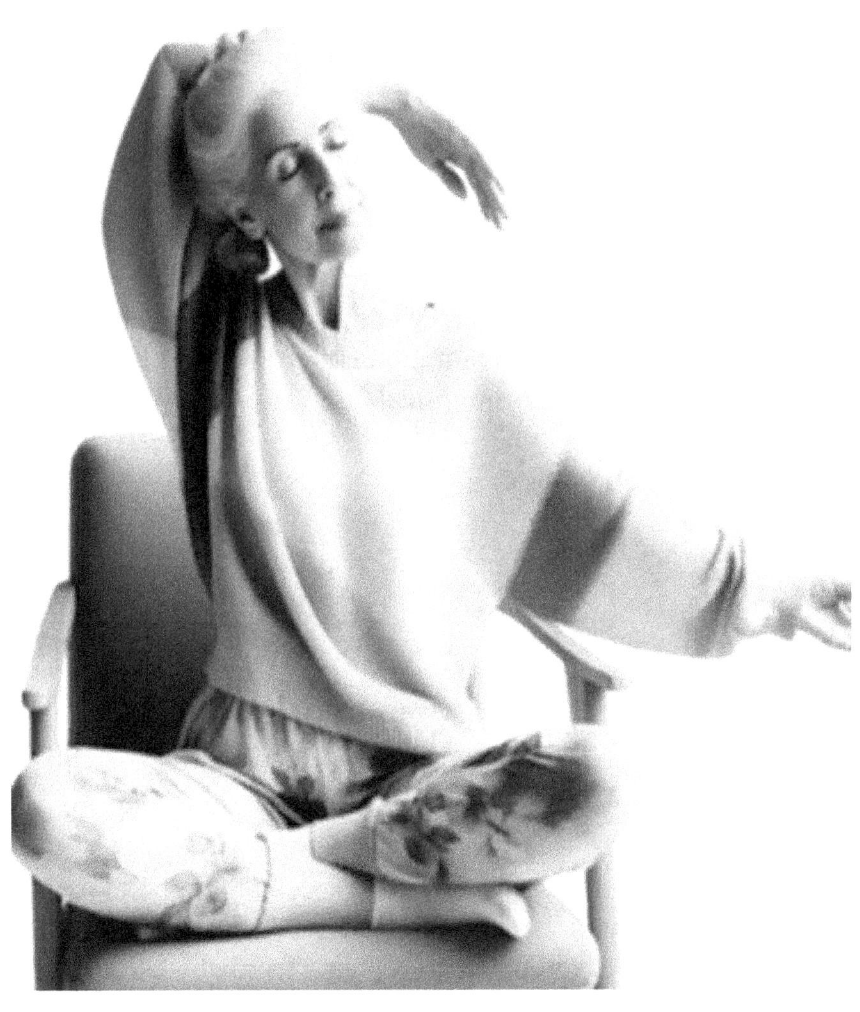

CHAPTER 3

Incorporating Diet for Holistic Health

In order to achieve holistic health, seniors must incorporate a well-rounded and healthy diet. Consider the Mediterranean diet as an example—an eating pattern known for improving general well-being via a mix of nutrient-rich foods and an emphasis on holistic health.

The Mediterranean Diet is distinguished by an abundance of fruits and vegetables, whole grains, legumes, nuts, seeds, and olive oil. It emphasizes lean proteins, particularly fish and fowl, and includes moderate dairy consumption, such as yogurt and cheese. This diet restricts the consumption of red meat and processed foods. A significant element is the use of red wine in moderation, usually during meals.

Key Elements:

- Fruits and vegetables are the cornerstone of the Mediterranean diet since they are high in vitamins, minerals, and antioxidants. They benefit heart health, immunological function, and supply critical nutrients for overall wellness.
- Olive oil, a mainstay in this diet, is a good source of monounsaturated fats. These fats are well-known for their heart-protective effects, as well as their contribution to cognitive wellness.
- Fatty fish, such as salmon and mackerel, are high in omega-3 fatty acids, which are essential for cardiovascular health and cognitive function. Lean proteins from chicken, lentils, and legumes supply necessary amino acids.

- Whole grains, such as brown rice, quinoa, and whole wheat, include complex carbs, fiber, and a variety of nutrients. They promote intestinal health and add to long-term energy levels.
- Moderate Dairy: Dairy products such as Greek yogurt and cheese include calcium, which is important for bone health. To reduce calorie and saturated fat consumption, the emphasis is on moderation.

Benefits of Holistic Health:

1. Cardiovascular Health: The Mediterranean diet has been linked to a lower risk of cardiovascular disease due to its emphasis on healthy fats, omega-3 fatty acids, and antioxidants.
2. Cognitive Function: Omega-3 fatty acid incorporation benefits cognitive health, perhaps lowering the risk of age-related cognitive decline.
3. Digestive Health: The high fiber component of the diet helps digestive health by reducing constipation and promoting a healthy gut microbiota.
4. Weight control: The Mediterranean diet assists in weight control by emphasizing complete, nutrient-dense meals, lowering the risk of obesity-related health concerns.

Remember that this is only a recommendation, not a strict score. Consult a healthcare practitioner to tailor your melody, including cultural favorites, allergies, and modifying to your specific requirements.

The Mediterranean diet is a philosophy of plenty and connection, not merely a set of rules. Cook with loved ones, enjoy fresh, seasonal ingredients, and celebrate the joy of cooking.

Listening to your body, practicing mindful eating, and working with a healthcare practitioner may help you turn your diet into a lively symphony of holistic health, one delicious note at a time.

So, start the music! Conduct your own personal health orchestra, enjoy the music of healthy cuisine, and revel in the bliss of overall well-being.

Introduction to Senior-Friendly Diet

As we age gracefully, our bodies whisper changes, and our nutritional demands respond to the quiet symphony of aging. Fear not, my friend; a senior-friendly diet is a celebration of wonderful, healthful food that feeds both your body and spirit.

Consider your plate to be a riot of color, with each mouthful a happy chorus of nutrients that support:

- **Strong Bones, Steady Steps**: Calcium and vitamin D take center stage, providing harmony to bone health. Dairy in all its creamy glory, leafy greens like kale and spinach, and even fortified meals join the band to keep your bones strong and your stride confident.
- **Muscle Melody, Sustained Strength**: While age may hint of muscle loss, protein sings a counterpoint. Lean meats, fish, eggs, and even plant-based proteins like beans and lentils join the chorus, helping you grow and retain muscle and stay strong and independent.
- **Cognitive Harmony, Memory's Maestro**: Forget about brain fog! Foods high in omega-3 fatty acids, antioxidants, and B vitamins, such as fatty fish, colorful fruits and vegetables, and whole grains, are included in a senior-friendly diet.

These nutrients partner with your cognitive function to maintain your memory bright and your intellect a lively conductor of daily life.

❖ **The Delicate Dance of Digestion:** As we become older, our gut health becomes a graceful waltz. Fiber takes the lead, facilitating regularity and nutritional absorption. It is found in whole grains, fruits, and vegetables. Probiotics, such as yogurt and fermented foods, contribute to the rhythm, keeping your digestive system joyfully humming.

❖ **Mindful Melodies, Joyful Bites**: Food is more than just nutrition; it's a celebration! Sharing meals with loved ones, enjoying every mouthful, and practicing mindful eating all contribute to a symphony of joy and connection. This emotional well-being feeds your soul and fuels a full existence.

Remember, there is no such thing as a one-size-fits-all senior diet. Consult a healthcare practitioner to tailor your nutritional composition to your specific requirements, tastes, and health problems.

Accept the delight of exploration, try new flavors, and heed to your body's whispers. A senior-friendly diet isn't a nuisance; it's a tasty, satisfying path to a healthier, happier you. Raise your fork, command the symphony of bright food, and enjoy the song of happiness in every mouthful.

Nutritional Tips for Energy and Recovery

Do you have a lethargic feeling? Slow to recover from workouts? Your body, like a high-performance engine, need the proper fuel and maintenance to function properly. Let's look at some dietary advice to boost your energy, improve your recuperation, and keep you going strong:

1. **Carbohydrates:** The Powerhouse: Consider carbs to be your fuel gauge. Choose complex carbs such as whole grains, fruits, and vegetables for long-lasting energy that does not spike your blood sugar. Refined carbohydrates, such as white bread and sweet pastries, provide a brief rush followed by a crash, leaving you feeling depleted.
2. **Protein:** The Foundation: Protein is your muscles' critical repair team. Within 2 hours of your activity, have 20-40 grams of protein (think lean meats, eggs, Greek yogurt, or plant-based options). This aids in the rebuilding of muscle tissue, minimizing discomfort and hastening recovery.
3. **Fats:** The Primary Lubricants: Don't be afraid of fat! Avocados, almonds, seeds, and olive oil include healthy fats that keep your engine working smoothly. They provide energy to your brain, help in hormone synthesis, and even aid in nutrient absorption. Healthy fats should be preferred over saturated and trans fats found in processed meals.
4. **The Vital Coolant:** Hydration Because your body is 60% water, staying hydrated is critical. Aim for 8-10 glasses of water each day, and significantly more during strenuous exercise or hot weather. Dehydration can sap your vitality and make recovery more difficult.
5. **Electrolytes as a Recharge Boost:** Sweating causes electrolytes such as salt, potassium, and magnesium to be lost during activity. To help in muscular function and reduce tiredness, replenish them with sports drinks, coconut water, or electrolyte pills.
6. **Pay Attention to Your Body:** Cravings might be messages from your body. Go for a salad if you're wanting greens! If you're craving something sweet, try a piece of fruit or a handful of almonds. Pay attention to your body's signals and give it what it requires, not simply what's on the menu.

7. **Mindful Eating**: Take your time eating, taste your meal, and avoid distractions. This aids digestion, increases satiety, and avoids overeating. It also allows you to reconnect with your body and make deliberate decisions about what you feed it.
8. **Don't Skip Meals:** Skipping meals can cause energy dumps and make recovery more difficult. To keep your energy levels steady and your metabolism revved up, aim for frequent meals and snacks throughout the day.
9. **Make Sleep a Priority:** Sleep is the ultimate rest break. Each night, aim for 7-8 hours of decent sleep. When you get enough sleep, your body has the energy it needs to function and recuperate at its best.

Food is more than simply food; it is also a source of joy, community, and well-being. Cook with loved ones, experiment with new dishes, and relish the sensation of mindful eating. This healthy eating relationship will nurture your body, mind, and soul.

Remember that your body is a one-of-a-kind engine. Experiment, pay attention to its murmurs, and provide it with the proper nutritional tools. These are simply suggestions; find out what works best for you and see your energy skyrocket as you recover with grace. So strap up, step on the throttle, and enjoy the trip!

"Wrinkles? Badges of wisdom. Aches? Whispers of change. Listen, adjust, keep dancing, age is just a song!"

CHAPTER 4

Positive Thinking and Motivation

Adopting low-impact exercise as a senior is more than simply a physical benefit; it's a beautiful dance with your body, fuelled by positive thinking and persistent motivation. These are the intangible wings that take you higher, making your adventure more bright and long-lasting.

Consider this: instead of dreading exercise, you view it as a lighthearted discovery of your abilities, a celebration of movement that generates delight. Every stride demonstrates your optimistic attitude, pulling you ahead with renewed zeal.

Positive thought serves as a vitamin for your low-impact journey. This is how it shines:

It reframes difficulties: aches and limits become possibilities for creative adjustments. "My knees aren't perfect?" is transformed into "Let's find water exercises I love!" This adjustment in viewpoint energizes you and keeps you moving.

It revels in minor victories: every step counts, and every stretch is a triumph. Positive thinking allows you to recognize and enjoy these minor victories, which fosters a sense of success and keeps you on course.

Positivity attracts cheerleaders because it is contagious. When you exude positivity, you draw the support and encouragement of loved ones as well as strangers. This sense of camaraderie boosts your motivation and creates a cheerful atmosphere around your workout regimen.

Motivation, or the fire in your heart, becomes the driving force behind your quest. Here are some stokers to keep it going:

- Set SMART objectives: Make your goals Specific, Measurable, Achievable, Relevant, and Time-bound. "Walk for 30 minutes twice a week" is more powerful than "Get more active."
- Discover your passion: Investigate several hobbies until you find what makes you happy. What is tai chi? Swimming? Dancing with your pals? Find out what sparks your inner flame and maintain it.
- Celebrate your accomplishments and reward yourself! After a good week, treat yourself to a spa day, get that new sportswear you've been eyeing, or organize a social trip with your fitness mates.
- Track your success: Using a diary or fitness apps helps you to visualize your accomplishments, inspiring pride and encouraging you to go farther.

Note, that positive thinking and motivation are both muscles that require workout. Practice thankfulness, focus on the joy of activity, and surround oneself with people who are encouraging. Your low-impact voyage will be light, happy, and sustainable with these invisible wings, bringing you to a future full of well-being and a grin on your face.

So, raise your head, bask in the sunshine of positivity, stoke the flames of inspiration, and take off on your one-of-a-kind low-impact trip. Every stride, every grin, every laugh demonstrates the power of a positive attitude and an unshakeable spirit. Move with fun and confidence, and watch your trip take off!

The Role of a Positive Mindset

Imagine traversing life's journey in golden sunlight, with every struggle greeted with optimism and every failure viewed as a springboard for progress. This is the power of a good attitude, my friend, a transformational force that transforms not only your ideas, but your whole world.

Consider your mind to be a lush garden. When good seeds like optimism, appreciation, and resilience are planted, beautiful blossoms of well-being emerge. These blossoms have an affect on every aspect of your life:

1. **Health in Balance**: Research shows a definite correlation between positive and physical health. A good attitude boosts your immune system, decreases stress, and promotes speedier healing. Consider approaching obstacles with calm, allowing optimism to increase your resilience and lead the way to higher well-being.
2. **Resilience Increases:** Life delivers curveballs, but a positive outlook permits you to recover gracefully. You view losses as chances to learn and grow rather than as a source of frustration. This inner strength serves as a shield, shielding you from negativity and fuelling your onward progress.
3. **Relationships Bloom**: Positivity spreads. Positive energy attracts like-minded individuals, building satisfying interactions and cultivating a supportive community. Imagine your days being filled with laughter, real friendships sprouting around you, and a sense of belonging enhancing your life.
4. **Productivity Soars:** Negativity drags you down, but optimism pushes you up. A positive mentality feeds your drive and motivation, increasing productivity and your capacity to achieve your objectives.

Consider yourself approaching work with zeal, creativity flowing easily, and success following as a natural result of your positive attitude.

5. **Joy, the Leading Light**: Positivity isn't only about strength and perseverance; it's also about appreciating the small victories. The pillars of a really meaningful existence are savoring life's basic pleasures, recognizing beauty in everyday moments, and finding joy in the journey.

Developing a good mentality is a process, not a destination. Here are some easy methods to cultivating your inner sunshine:

- Practice gratitude: Think on something you're grateful for, even if it's tiny. Keep a gratitude notebook or express your thankfulness to loved ones.
- Negative ideas should be challenged: identify and reframe gloomy thoughts as opportunities or lessons learnt.
- Mindfulness methods such as meditation can assist you in anchoring yourself in the present moment, appreciating it without succumbing to stress or regret.
- Surround yourself with individuals who are upbeat: Seek out folks that raise you up and inspire you, and build a supporting network to feed your positivity.
- Small wins should be celebrated: Recognize and appreciate your accomplishments, no matter how minor. Every step closer to your goals is a reason for celebration.

Remember that having a good mentality does not mean disregarding reality; it means selecting your perspective. You may convert your life into a bright narrative of resilience, joy, and limitless possibilities with intentional work and a dedication to creating inner sunlight.

So, let your optimism serve as a compass, and your pleasure serve as a guiding light, and watch your life blossom with each step you take on your positive path.

Accept the sunshine from inside and watch your world flourish!

Motivational Stories and Strategies

Adopting low-impact exercise as a senior is more than simply physical movement; it is a dynamic dance with life, inspired by inspiring tales and effective tactics. Let us enter this realm of delicate strength and pleasant movement!

1. **Motivational Songs**: Consider the Grandma Runner. Harriette Thompson, 86, is elegantly conquering marathons and showing that age is only a number. "No limits, just possibilities!" her narrative exclaims.
2. **The Chair Yoga Guru**: Consider Fred Devito, who has turned his retirement into a journey of strength and flexibility via chair yoga. "Movement comes in all forms, find yours!" he says.
3. **The Dancing Couple**: See Dorothy, 93, and Bill, 95, tapping their way to happiness! "Joy fuels movement," their narrative tells us. "Move to the rhythm of your heart."

Strategies for Implementation:

- Begin with simply 10 minutes of walking and progressively increase the time and effort. Each step is a success, and each day marks a new milestone on your journey.
- Discover Your Groove: Consider trying water aerobics, tai chi, chair yoga, or dance. Discover the activity that brings out your inner DJ and makes you want to dance.

- Companionship: Traveling with friends or family offers fun, support, and accountability. Find your exercising rhythm with your favorite workout buddies.
- Music is Magic: Make a playlist that raises your spirits and gets you moving. Allow the rhythm to guide your steps and the rich colors of music to paint your exercise.
- Keep Track of Your Successes: To track your progress, keep a notebook or use a fitness app. Seeing your accomplishments, no matter how large or tiny, boosts inspiration and keeps you on course.

Remember that your low-impact path is a one-of-a-kind tune. Choose tales that speak to your soul, put techniques in place that work for you, and most all, enjoy the song of movement. Every stride, every bend, every laugh - these are the notes that make up your wonderful symphony of well-being.

So put on your walking shoes, turn on some music, and let the tales and ideas encourage you to move with confidence, grace, and a grin. Every senior has the capacity to become a low-impact exercise maestro, a song of strength and joy resonating down the years. Accept your rhythm, walk with purpose, and watch your life bloom with vivid health and pleasure!

Maintaining Enthusiasm Throughout the Journey

As a senior, engaging in low-impact exercise is more than simply a physical adventure; it's a dynamic dance with life, fuelled by unrelenting excitement. But, let's face it, even the most enthusiastic dancers require an energy boost from time to time. Here are some pointers to keep the fire burning during your low-impact journey:

1. Change it Up: Routine may be the enemy of excitement. Change up your walking route, attend a different tai chi class,

or even go swimming! Variety keeps your mind and body engaged, preventing "been-there-done-that" syndrome.

2. Embrace Nature's Symphony: Get away from the gym walls and immerse yourself in nature's colorful song. Walk beneath rustling leaves, breathe in the fresh air, and feel the sun on your skin. The beauty of nature energizes your spirit and provides a wonderful touch to your movement.

3. Laughter is Important: Sharing the trip with loved ones increases the delight. Find a workout partner or join a senior fitness group. Laughter, discussion, and triumphs shared become the unseen wind that pulls you onward.

4. Rejoice in Small Victories: Do not wait for marathon medals to rejoice! Recognize every set done, every additional lap walked, and every agony endured. These apparently minor successes are stepping stones to your happiness and ought to be celebrated.

5. Fuel Your Movement: Your food choices have an influence on your energy levels. Feed your body nutritious fats, lean protein, and colorful fruits and veggies. A well-fueled body moves more easily and enthusiastically.

6. Monitor Your Progress: Seeing your accomplishments boosts your confidence and keeps you motivated. Keep a notebook, utilize a fitness app, or capture images of your progress. Seeing your adventure unfold ignites your excitement and motivates you to keep going.

7. Reward Yourself: Recognize your hard work! After a good week, treat yourself to a spa day, purchase that new water bottle you've been eyeing, or schedule a picnic with your fitness mates. Rewards make the trip more enjoyable and remind you of the importance you place on your well-being.

8. Discover Your Passion: Low-impact exercise should not be a chore. Find an activity that brings out your inner kid, whether it's dancing with pals or perfecting chair yoga positions. Passion fuels excitement and turns action into a joyous celebration.

9. Concentrate on the Joy: It's not about climbing Everest; it's about dancing with life. Concentrate on the pleasure of movement, the power you're acquiring, and the freedom you're obtaining. Allow the good feelings to fuel your excitement and brighten your journey.

10. Rejoice Every Day: Life is a priceless gift. Accept each exercise, stroll, and stretch as a celebration of your body and spirit. Gratitude and gratitude keep the fire burning, making each step a monument to your dynamic path.

Maintaining excitement is a journey rather than a destination. Accept these suggestions, listen to your body, and, most importantly, have fun! Your low-impact trip is one-of-a-kind, full of personal victories and pleasant moments. Move with passion, rejoice in minor successes, and watch your zeal illuminate the way to a lively and meaningful existence.

So put on your dance shoes, turn on your favorite music, and follow the beat of your heart. Remember, a senior dancer is a force to be reckoned with, exuding energy and motivating others to engage in the joyful song of well-being. Keep moving, laughing, and the fire burning!

CHAPTER 5

Step-by-Step Exercise Guides

Adopting low-impact exercise as a senior is more than simply physical movement; it's a dynamic dance with life, powered by the assurance that you know what to do! Fear not, seasoned explorer; these step-by-step instructions will turn your excursion into a lovely dance of well-being:

<u>Chair Yoga Symphony</u>

- Locate your center: Sit up straight on a firm chair, your feet level on the floor. Deeply inhale, feeling your spine extend and shoulders unfold. This is your anchor, your resting position.
- Raise your arms upward, palms facing each other, for the Sunrise Stretch. Consider reaching for the sun in the morning. Feel your chest expand and your neck lengthen. Hold for 5 seconds.
- Twirling the Twinkling Stars: Looking over your shoulder, gently shift your body to one side. Deeply inhale, feeling your spine twist and stretch. Rep on the opposite side. Each hold for 5 seconds.
- Tranquility Tree stance: Place one foot on the opposing knee to form a "tree" stance. Balance and focus on your core while you ground your standing leg. Hold for 10 breaths, seeking calm in the midst of motion.

Relaxation and Roll your shoulders and wrists gently, then breathe deeply. Celebrate the completion of your movement symphony, a happy song for your well-being.

Walking Oasis on the Water:

- Enter the rejuvenating haven: Search for a shallow pool or a water aerobics class. Begin by wading comfortably, taking use of the water's buoyancy and support. Imagine yourself dancing with mermaids!
- Marching Rhythms: Take rhythmic forward steps with your knees slightly elevated and your arms swinging at your sides. Feel the resistance of the water tone your legs and chill your body.
- Arm Circles for Happy Armadillos Extend your arms to the sides and move them in gentle, circular strokes, palms down. Consider making bubbles with your fingertips in the water.
- Lift your knees up one at a time, bringing your thighs towards your chest. Engage your core while allowing the water to massage your legs. Allow the hilarity to erupt!
- Float and reflect: Lean back gently and float on your back, allowing the water to embrace your entire body. Close your eyes and let the peace to wash over you.

Graceful Tai Chi Melodies

- Locate your center: Stand with your feet hip-width apart, knees slightly bent, and arms at your sides, relaxed. Close your eyes and concentrate on your breathing. This is your anchor note.
- Raise your arms upward, palms facing each other, to embrace the Willow Tree. Consider swinging lightly in the breeze like a willow. Feel your spine lengthening and your chest opening. Hold for 5 seconds.
- Gentle Flow Steps: Step forward with one foot, gradually transferring your weight and lowering your center of

gravity. Rep with the opposite foot. Move in time with your breathing.

- To open and close the sky, extend one arm to the side, palm down, then gently arc it overhead, palm up. Rep on the opposite side. Imagine your beautiful movements expanding and shutting the sky.
- Circle the Moon: With both arms in front of you, draw slow, little circles, one clockwise and the other counterclockwise. Concentrate on your breathing and relax your arms.

Remember, these are only guiding notes; you may tailor them to your own rhythm and tastes. Listen to your body, make adjustments as required, and most importantly, dance with delight! Each step is a note in your well-being symphony, creating a vivid song of health and happiness.

So put on your dance shoes (or comfy clothing!), locate a sunny area, and let these step-by-step instructions lead the way. You create a masterpiece of vibrant life with every movement and breath. Accept the delight, move confidently, and enjoy the rhythm of your own one-of-a-kind low-impact journey!

Introduction to Low-Impact Exercises

Adopting low-impact exercise as a senior is more than just ticking a box on a doctor's appointment; it's about kindling a lively dance with life, full of joy, strength, and limitless possibilities. Forget about treadmills and heavy weights; this trip unfolds in softer rhythms, when exercise becomes a celebration of your health.

Let's take a look at why low-impact workouts are ideal dance partners:

- Gentle yet powerful: No hammering or jarring, simply gentle, controlled motions that build your muscles and improve your balance. Consider shaping your body in the manner of a skilled potter, using soft touches and deliberate intentions.
- Open the Door to Joy: Let go of the struggle and embrace the joy! Chair yoga, water walking, and tai chi are all low-impact workouts disguised as joyful dances. As you move with friends, connect with your inner child, and experience the sheer joy of mindful movement, laughter will rise up.
- Fuel Your Wellbeing Symphony: Every step, stretch, and elegant movement becomes a note in your well-being symphony. Increase your energy, sleep better, and feel your mood improve as you exercise your body and nurture your spirit.
- A Universe of Possibilities: Don't be a wallflower at this lively party! There's something for everyone, from the rhythmic steps of water walking to the flowing melodies of tai chi. Discover your ideal fit via swimming, dancing, light weight exercise, or even gardening.
- Begin Small, Dream Big: This symphony does not require a spectacular beginning; instead, begin with a soft hum. Begin by walking for 10 minutes and progressively increase the time and intensity as you establish your rhythm. Every stride is a win, and every session is a climax of happiness.
- You are the conductor of your own movement symphony, so pay attention to your body. Adjust workouts as required, take pauses as needed, and appreciate your own pace. This journey is all about listening to and honoring your body's wisdom.
- Find Your Tribe and Spread the Joy! Exercising with friends, joining a senior fitness club, or finding a supportive

spouse are all options. Laughter, discussion, and shared victories feed your motivation and build a thriving community that supports you.

- Fuel Your Movement: Feed your body healthy nutrients to keep your energy levels up and your body in tune. Consider colorful fruits and veggies, lean protein, and healthy fats - a delectable symphony powering your joyous movement.

- Celebrate Every Victory: Don't wait for the grand finale; celebrate every note! Recognize your progress, no matter how minor. Every set done, every additional lap completed, and every soreness endured is a testimonial to your effort and merits a pleased nod.

- Remember that low-impact exercise is a dynamic invitation to dance with life, not a duty. Put on your most comfortable clothing, turn on your favorite music, and enter the arena of your own well-being. You create a masterpiece of vivid life with each beautiful movement and happy laugh. Accept the beat, walk confidently, and watch your trip unfold into a symphony of joy and wellness!

- So, lovely senior explorer, are you ready to dance? A song of possibilities awaits in the form of low-impact workout. Step onto the stage with an open heart and a fun attitude, release your inner dancer, and create your own bright symphony of well-being!

Detailed Instructions and Proper Form

It is important to move with intention before embarking on your low-impact path. Let's get into the specifics, emphasizing exact directions and appropriate form to guarantee your travel is not only enjoyable but also safe and effective:

1. Flow of Chair Yoga: Sit tall with your feet firmly on the floor, spine straight, and shoulders relaxed in Mountain Pose. Engage your core, stretch your neck, and take deep breaths. (5 deep breathes)

- Tree stance: Lift one foot gently and place it on the opposing knee to form a "tree" stance. Breathe steadily and evenly for 10 breaths. Rep on the opposite side.
  Extend your arms to the sides, parallel to the floor, palms facing down. Cross your forearms in front of your chest, fingers pointing to the ceiling. Hold for 5 seconds.
  Come onto your hands and knees, with your hands shoulder-width apart and your knees hip-width apart. Inhale deeply while arching your back and gazing up like a cat. Exhale with a cow-like rounding of the back and tucking of the chin. Rep 5 times more.

2. Walking Oasis on the Water: Wading Serenity: Enter the pool slowly, experiencing the buoyancy and support of the water. Begin by swimming comfortably, taking modest steps, and slowly swinging your arms at your sides. (three minutes)

- Marching Mermaid: Move forward in rhythmic steps, keeping your upper body relaxed and your arms swinging at your sides. As you march, feel the water's resistance cool your legs. (three minutes)
- Arm Circles for Laughter: Extend your arms to the sides and move them in gentle, circular strokes, palms down. Consider making fun bubbles in the water. (Two minutes)
  Lift your knees up one at a time, bringing your thighs towards your chest. Engage your core while allowing the water to massage your legs. Allow the hilarity to erupt! (Two minutes)

3. Graceful Tai Chi Melodies: Stand with your feet hip-width apart, knees slightly bent, and arms relaxed at your sides. Close your eyes and center yourself by focusing on your breath.

- Allow the Sky to Open: Raise one arm slowly to the side, palm down, then arc it overhead, palm up. Rep on the opposite side, feeling your chest open and your spine extend. (5 deep breaths on each side)
- Gentle Flow Steps: Step forward with one foot, gradually transferring your weight and lowering your center of gravity. Rep with the opposite foot, moving in time with your breath.
  Stand with your feet together and your knees slightly bent to embrace the Willow. Lean forward from your hips, keeping your back straight, and hang your arms freely. Consider swinging lightly in the breeze like a willow tree. (5 deep breathes)

Formal Guidelines:

- Listen to your body: Modify workouts as appropriate and take breaks as needed.
- Engage your core: For appropriate posture and stability, keep your abdominal muscles slightly pushed in.
- Controlled movement: Avoid jerky motions and instead concentrate on smooth, thoughtful transitions.
- Maintain proper posture: Maintain a straight spine, relaxed shoulders, and a raised chin.
- Breathe deeply: Throughout the exercises, focus on your breath to stay calm and energized.

If you experience any pain, stop immediately and inform your doctor.

Remember, these are only suggestions; listen to your body, experiment with different options, and most importantly, have fun!

Your low-impact journey is a celebration of your body and its possibilities, not a competition. Move with elegance and delight, and watch your well-being flourish as you create your own bright masterpiece of health and happiness.

So, go into the intricacies, perfect your form, and dance confidently! Allow each walk, stretch, and conscious breath to be a testimonial to your commitment and a happy song in your symphony of well-being!

Gradual Progression Plans

Your low-impact workout adventure is about more than simply putting your toes in the water; it's about overcoming calm oceans and uncovering secret coral reefs: vivid possibilities just waiting to be discovered. But how can you traverse these waters in a safe and successful manner? Gradual progression plans are your map and compass, leading you with each gentle step toward increased strength, flexibility, and joy.

Consider this: You begin with 10 minutes of chair yoga, feeling the sun on your skin as your muscles stretch. You add 5 minutes a week later, feeling stronger and more confident. This is the core of slow growth, my friend: tiny, sustainable gains that lead to huge long-term consequences.

Why are these plans so important?

Injury prevention: By gradually increasing the intensity and length, you allow your body to adjust and avoid overexertion.

Boost your self-esteem: Seeing your success, no matter how modest, keeps you motivated and dancing with delight.

Continue to be challenged: As your body changes, so should your strategy, ensuring that you continue to get the advantages of activity.

Customized for you: No two travels are same. Your strategy should take into account your preferences, fitness level, and any physical constraints.

Let's look at some examples of advancement plans:

Flow of Chair Yoga:

- **Week 1:** 10 minutes of fundamental positions such as mountain pose, tree pose, and mild stretches.
- **Week 2:** Add 5 minutes of arm balances and twists.
- **Week 3**: Concentrate on deeper stretches and holding each position for extended periods of time.
- **Week 4:** Experiment with different variants of common positions and incorporate a brief sequence of standing motions.

Walking Oasis on the Water:

Week 1: 10 minutes of wading and shallow walking, with an emphasis on balance and coordination.

Week 2: Add 5 minutes of marching steps and arm circles to your routine.

Week 3: Begin incorporating high knees and mild leg lifts.

Week 4: Intensify your motions and try short laps around the pool.

Graceful Tai Chi Melodies

Week 1: Concentrate on fundamental postures such as standing meditation and opening and shutting the sky.

Week 2: Incorporate slow, flowing movements, such as willow tree sways and gradual walks.

Week 3: Include arm circles and balancing exercises.

Week 4: Try out more intricate sequences while focusing on keeping smooth, beautiful motions.

Remember that these are only samples. Consult your doctor before beginning any workout program, and don't be afraid to change or tweak the plans to meet your specific needs. Pay attention to your body, rejoice in your accomplishments, and keep moving with enthusiasm!

Gradual growth is about relishing the trip, one patient step at a time, rather than racing to the finish line. You strengthen your body, nurture your spirit, and create your own masterpiece of bright well-being with each movement. So, unfold your map, accept the gentle stream, and let your slow growth plan to lead you to a life full of happy movement and limitless possibilities!

Guidance on Designing a Tailored Routine

Adopting low-impact exercise as a senior isn't a one-size-fits-all solution; it's about creating your own joyous symphony of movement, adapted to your individual rhythm and goals.

Forget the cookie-cutter plans, and instead dive into the art of creating a routine that honors your uniqueness while also fueling your well-being at every step.

- **Hear Your Preferences' Melody:** What stirs your spirit? Do you long for tai chi's soft swing, water walking's rhythmic delight, or chair yoga's meditative flow? Choose activities that pique your inner dancer and keep your pulse pounding with excitement.
- **Pay attention to your body:** Are there any workouts that make you feel weird or uneasy? Take note of your physical limitations and adapt or replace techniques as necessary. This isn't a race; it's a celebration of your body's distinct qualities. Can you commit to 30 minutes of activity every day, or do you prefer shorter bursts of movement? Create a program with realistic lengths and time limits that fit into your life.
- **Align with Your Wellbeing Objectives:** Looking for strength and balance? Exercises that use your core muscles and challenge your coordination, such as chair squats, arm circles, and the flowing motions of tai chi, should be prioritized.

Do you want to be more flexible and relaxed? Gentle stretches, yoga positions such as cat-cow, and deep breathing exercises will become your soothing song, melting away stress and increasing the suppleness of your body.

Do you yearn for a social routine? Join a group class, pair up with a friend, or even join an online community to find joy. Sharing the trip with others adds a bright symphony of shared victories, as well as laughter and support.

Improve Your Movement Symphony: Begin small, but dream big: Don't put yourself through a long workout program.

Begin with 10-15 minutes of exercise every day and progressively increase the time and intensity as your body adjusts and your confidence grows.

Keep your routine interesting by varying it! Experiment with new activities, try new variants on old favorites, and add a dash of spontaneity to keep your movement symphony fresh and exciting.

Music has the power to transform: Play your favorite music! Allow the beat to direct your feet, boost your enthusiasm, and paint your workout in the brilliant colors of your musical preferences.

Keep track of your progress: Celebrate your accomplishments, no matter how tiny! Keep a notebook, utilize a fitness app, or capture images of your progress. Seeing your adventure unfold keeps you motivated and dancing with delight.

Remember that your personalized regimen is a living song that changes with you, not a strict script. Listen to your body, accept the joy of movement, and don't be afraid to change the notes as you go. This is your well-being symphony, and you're the conductor!

So put on your favorite comfy clothing, turn on your favorite music, and go onto the stage of your own colorful life. Embrace the rhythm of your individual tastes, listen to your body's suggestions, and allow your customized regimen become a joyous monument to your devotion and enthusiasm for life. Every stride, stretch, and movement contributes to your symphony of well-being, resulting in a masterpiece of vivid health and pleasure. Dance confidently, enjoy your uniqueness, and let the melody of your life lead you to a symphony of happy movement!

Setting Realistic Goals

Embracing low-impact fitness as a senior does not imply climbing Everest; rather, it entails enjoyable excursions with stunning views and sun-kissed lunches at the summit. Forget the strain of unachievable heights; instead, let's create realistic objectives that will feed your drive, celebrate your progress, and paint a bright picture of your well-being.

Why is it vital to set realistic goals?

- **Avoid discouragement:** Reaching for the moon might result in a painful landing. Setting attainable objectives boosts confidence and keeps you dancing through life.
- **Celebrate minor successes.** Witnessing development, no matter how modest, becomes a joyful song that fuels your urge to continue forward and explore.
- **Stay on track.** Unrealistic objectives are like mirages in the desert; they look promising but leave you thirsty. Setting reasonable goals keeps you motivated and moving ahead.
- **Tailored for you:** Your trip is unique. Your objectives should be based on your tastes, fitness level, and physical constraints.

Let's look at some practical goal-setting tips:

1. **Start small and dream big**: Begin with basic objectives, such as "walk for 10 minutes three times a week" or "do 5 gentle stretches in the morning." As your confidence grows, gently increase the length or intensity.
2. **Focus on the process rather than the outcome**: Don't only focus on decreasing weight or developing flexibility. Celebrate the joy of movement, the strength you're developing, and the peace you nurture.

3. **Listen to your body**. Be aware of your energy levels and physical limitations. Adjust your goals as appropriate, and prioritize rest and recuperation.
4. **Make it entertaining.** Select activities that you actually enjoy. Dancing, water walking, chair yoga - discover workouts that awaken your inner kid and keep you wanting more.
5. **Track your progress and celebrate your achievements!** Keep a notebook, utilize a fitness app, or capture images of your progress. Seeing your adventure develop motivates you and reminds you of how far you've come.

Remember that realistic objectives aren't about pushing yourself to your limits; they're about discovering sustainable methods to move your body and nourish your spirit.

Here are some examples of achievable, low-impact goals:

- Increase your walking time by 5 minutes every week.
- In one month, you'll be able to master three new chair yoga positions.
- Join a water aerobics class once a week.
- Stand on one leg for 30 seconds to improve your balance.
- Reduce your overall screen usage by 30 minutes each day, and utilize that time for easy stretching.
- Accept your uniqueness, listen to your body, and appreciate tiny successes. Your low-impact trip isn't a race; it's a passionate dance with life, complete with magnificent scenery and wonderful moments. Set reasonable goals that will influence your actions, not dictate them. With each delicate movement, you create your own masterpiece of well-being, a monument to your devotion and own rhythm of delight.

So put on your comfy shoes, turn on your favorite music, and take the first step on your sun-kissed walk. Conquering mountains isn't always about getting to the top; it's about enjoying the route, the laughing with friends, and the stunning views of your own bright well-being. Set attainable objectives, appreciate minor triumphs, and dance with life to the beat of your delight!

Sample Workout Plans for Different Levels and Time Commitments

Embracing low-impact exercise as a senior is a colorful symphony in which everyone dances to their own beat. Whether you're a seasoned maestro or a newbie pounding your toes, a beautiful movement melody awaits you. Let's look at some sample workout regimens to boost your well-being, regardless of your ability or time commitment:

- The "Sunrise Serenade" - Beginner (15 minutes):
- Gentle Greeting: Begin with 5 minutes of focused breathing and mild stretches like arm circles and neck rolls.
- Flowing Harmony: Transition to 5 minutes of chair yoga, concentrating on fundamental positions such as mountain pose, tree pose, and sitting twist.
- Cool-down Crescendo: Finish with 5 minutes of relaxing stretches, such as reclining down and focusing on deep breathing.
- The "Midday Movement" - Intermediate (30 minutes):
- Energizing Warm up: Begin with 10 minutes of quick walking, marching in place, or light water aerobics.
- Strengthening Symphony: Perform 10 minutes of seated or standing movements with small weights, focusing on squats, lunges, and bicep curls.

- Flexibility Finish: Cool down with 10 minutes of moderate stretches such as cat-cow, hamstring, and chest openers.
- The "Sunset Soiree" - Advanced (45 minutes)
- Invigorating Overture: Begin with 15 minutes of vigorous walking, followed by Tai Chi moves such as swaying willow trees and opening and closing the sky.
- balancing Ballet: Begin with 15 minutes of balancing exercises such as standing on one leg, heel-toe walking, and easy yoga positions like Warrior III.
- Strength and Flexibility Encore: Finish with 15 minutes of strength training with resistance bands or bodyweight movements, followed by deeper stretches such as butterfly posture and forward fold. Remember, these are only beginning points!
- Adjust time and intensity: As you develop confidence, listen to your body and alter or extend your workouts.
- Mix and combine activities. Create your own symphony by mixing workouts from different levels or including your favorite low-impact hobbies.
- Concentrate on the thrill of movement: Avoid getting caught up in counting reps or chasing numbers. Celebrate the sensation of moving your body and appreciate the experience.
- Find Your Tribe: Join a group fitness class, work out with a friend, or connect with an online community. Sharing the trip brings humor, motivation, and a lively song of shared victories.

Your Low-Impact trip is a blank canvas, waiting to be painted with bright strokes of movement and delight. Choose your colors, discover your rhythm, and create your own masterpiece of well-being. With each step, you create a symphony of strength, flexibility, and enjoyment, demonstrating that age is only a number in the dance of life. So put on your comfy clothing, turn on your favorite music, and let the songs of movement lead you to a joyous, vivid existence!

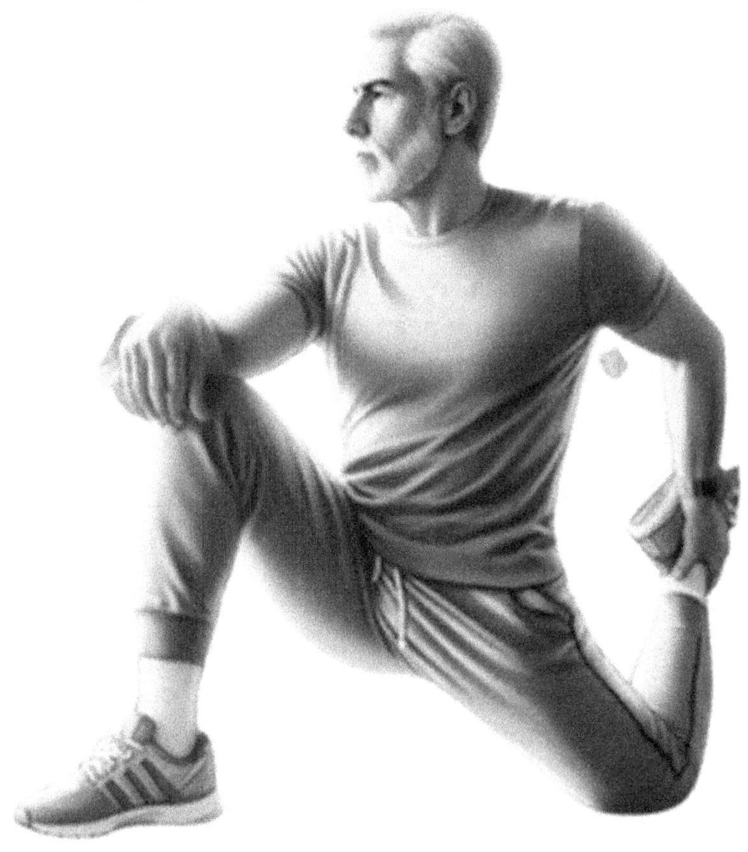

CHAPTER 7

Dos and Don'ts for Safe Exercise

Embracing low-impact exercise as a senior isn't just about moving your body; it's about dancing with life safely and joyfully, with every step a graceful note in your symphony of well-being. But to truly revel in the rhythm, it's important to understand the do's and don'ts of safe movement. So, put on your comfortable shoes, and let's explore the harmonious path to joyful, injury-free exercise!

Do...:

1. Listen to your body: Your body whispers wisdom; pay attention! Stop or modify exercises if you feel pain, discomfort, or dizziness.
2. Warm up and cool down: Gently prepare your muscles with 5-10 minutes of light movement before your workout, and wind down with stretches afterwards.
3. Embrace proper form: Focus on posture, alignment, and controlled movements. Don't force anything; let grace guide your steps.
4. Stay hydrated: Drink plenty of water before, during, and after your exercise to keep your body lubricated and energized.
5. Wear comfortable clothes and shoes: Choose supportive shoes with good shock absorption and clothes that allow for free movement.
6. Choose activities you enjoy: Find low-impact exercises that spark your inner child, like water walking, chair yoga, or dancing. Joy fuels motivation and keeps you moving.
7. Listen to your doctor: Consult your doctor before starting any new exercise program, especially if you have any health concerns.

8. Modify and adapt: Don't be afraid to adjust exercises to suit your limitations and preferences. Your journey is unique, find your perfect rhythm.
9. Celebrate small victories: Witnessing progress, no matter how small, fuels your confidence and keeps you dancing with life.
10. Have fun! Laughter and joy are music to your body's ears. Let the movement feel playful and lighthearted.

Don't...:

1. Push yourself too hard: Listen to your body's signals and avoid overexertion. Leave the marathon training for younger souls.
2. Ignore pain: Pain is a warning sign; stop if you feel anything sharp or persistent. Consult your doctor if necessary.
3. Use heavy weights or risky equipment: Stick to light weights and exercises that maintain proper form and balance.
4. Move with jerky motions: Embrace smooth, controlled movements to avoid injuries.
5. Exercise on slippery surfaces: Choose safe exercise environments with good traction to prevent falls.
6. Hold your breath: Focus on breathing deeply and rhythmically throughout your workout.
7. Compare yourself to others: Your journey is yours alone. Celebrate your own progress and uniqueness.
8. Skip rest days: Your body needs time to recover. Schedule rest days to prevent fatigue and injuries.
9. Forget to have fun! Exercise should be a joyful experience. If it feels like a chore, find something else you love to do.

Remember, safe exercise isn't about restrictions; it's about creating a foundation for joyful movement and vibrant well-being. By staying informed, listening to your body, and prioritizing fun, you can compose a symphony of safe, joyful exercise that keeps you dancing with life for years to come.

So, put on your favorite tunes, take a deep breath, and step onto the stage of your own vibrant life. With every safe, graceful movement, you paint a masterpiece of health and happiness, proving that age is just a number in the beautiful dance of life. Dance with care, dance with joy, and create your own symphony of safe, joyful movement!

Safety Precautions and Warm-up Techniques

Stepping into the realm of low-impact fitness is more than just taking delicate steps in the sunshine; it's about dancing confidently and carefully with life. To properly enjoy the beat, however, understanding safety considerations and correct warm-up procedures is essential. It's similar like tuning your instrument before the symphony begins, ensuring that every note of movement resonates with happiness and well-being.

Safety First:

- Consult your doctor. Before starting any new workout regimen, especially if you have any health issues, see your doctor. They can direct you to activities that are safe and useful to you.
- Listen to your body. Your body is whispering knowledge; pay heed! Stop if you have any pain, dizziness, or discomfort. Pushing through can cause harm.
- Hydration represents harmony: Drinking enough of water before, during, and after exercise will keep your body lubricated and invigorated.

- Dress for the dance: Choose comfortable garments that allow for mobility and supportive shoes with high shock absorption. Safety should not come at the expense of elegance!
- Be mindful of your surroundings: Choose safe exercising surroundings with excellent traction to avoid falls. Uneven surfaces and slippery flooring are unwanted additions to your movement symphony.

Warm-Up Melodies:

- Gentle Greeting: Begin with 5-10 minutes of mild activity to wake up your muscles and joints. Consider gentle walking, arm circles, and neck rolls.
- Flowing Harmony: Use mild stretches to develop flexibility and prepare your body for movement. Concentrate on key muscular groups, such as your legs, back, and shoulders.
- Heartbeat In Tune: Gradually raise your heart rate with simple aerobic workouts such as jumping jacks (adjusted as appropriate), marching in place, or easy water walking.
- Remember that warm-ups aren't races; they're conversations with your body. Listen to its murmurs, adapt your motions as necessary, and let the beat lead you.

Bonus Tips:

- Buddy up! Exercising with a friend or taking a group class increases motivation and social contact, strengthening your safety net even further.
- Embrace fun! Laughter is the best medicine, so select things that you truly like. Movement that brings delight keeps you dancing with life.

- Celebrate minor successes. Witnessing improvement, no matter how tiny, boosts confidence and keeps you pushing forward.

Safety measures and warm-up practices are the first steps in creating a symphony of enjoyable, injury-free exercise. Making them a part of your movement routine establishes a foundation for well-being and confidence, allowing you to dance with life without worry. So put on your comfy shoes, turn on your favorite music, and stroll onto the stage of vivid movement. With each safe, attentive step, you build a masterpiece of health and pleasure, demonstrating that age is only a number in the wonderful dance of life. Dance with care and delight, and let the song of your well-being fill the air!

Common Mistakes to Avoid

Embracing low-impact exercise as a senior is more than just taking slow steps in the sunshine; it is about dancing with life with bright enthusiasm. However, to properly grasp this beautiful dance, it's vital to avoid certain frequent pitfalls that might impair your well-being:

- ❖ Ignoring Pain: Pain is a warning sign, not a willing dancing partner. If you are experiencing discomfort, stop immediately and adapt the activity or take a rest. Pushing through might result in injuries that keep you from enjoying your favorite activities.
- ❖ Pushing Too Hard: Recognize your body's boundaries. Don't try to run a marathon while your heart is singing the song of a slow waltz. To avoid overexertion and exhaustion, gradually increase both intensity and duration.

- ❖ Ignoring Proper Form: Sloppy movements may feel simpler, but they can cause muscular imbalances and discomfort. Concentrate on posture, alignment, and controlled motions. Remember that delicate steps result in a more beautiful symphony.
- ❖ Skipping the Warm-up: Think of your warm-up as tuning your instrument before you play. Gentle stretches and gentle activity prepare your muscles and joints to avoid strains and injuries.
- ❖ Forgetting to Hydrate: Your body, like plants, requires water to function properly. Stay hydrated before, during, and after your workout to keep your energy levels up and your body lubricated.
- ❖ Wearing the Wrong Gear: Uncomfortable clothing and shoes can transform your ecstasy into a waltz of frustration. Choose comfortable clothing and shoes with adequate shock absorption. Style and safety may make a beautiful duo!
- ❖ Comparing Yourself to Others: Each path is unique, with its own rhythm and pace. Avoid the mistake of comparing your leisurely walk to someone else's brisk salsa. Celebrate your own accomplishments and accept your uniqueness.
- ❖ Skipping rest days: Your body requires time to heal and rejuvenate. Schedule rest days to avoid muscular exhaustion and injury. Remember that rest is not stillness, but rather a quiet note in the song of your well-being.
- ❖ Forgetting to Have Fun: Movement should provide delight, not dread. Choose things that you really love, such as water walking, chair yoga, or dancing. Laughter and fun keep you motivated and pushing on with a positive attitude.

❖ Ignoring Your Doctor: Before beginning any new workout regimen, particularly if you have health concerns, consult your doctor. They can direct you toward safe and useful activities that meet your specific requirements.

Remember, avoiding these frequent mistakes isn't about establishing a rigid regimen; it's about laying the groundwork for happy, safe exercise. Listen to your body, practice mindfulness, and allow the rhythm of your health lead you. With each exquisite stride, you create a masterpiece of vigorous health and pleasure, demonstrating that age is only a number in the wonderful dance of life. So, put on your comfy shoes, turn on your favorite music, and take to the stage for your own enjoyable exercise trip!

Tips for Injury Prevention and Recovery

Embracing low-impact exercise as a senior is more than just taking light steps in the sunshine; it is about dancing with life with bright joy, free of the fear of injury. However, even elegant motions might be hampered by obstacles. To maintain your symphony of well-being singing pleasant notes, here are some injury prevention and rehabilitation methods.

Prevention Is the Best Medicine

1. Listen to Your Body: Your body speaks wisdom; pay heed! Stop or adjust workouts if you experience pain, discomfort, or dizziness. Pushing through might result in injuries that keep you from enjoying your favorite activities.
2. Respect proper form. Sloppy actions may feel easy, but they can cause muscular imbalances and discomfort.

Concentrate on posture, alignment, and controlled motions. Remember that delicate steps result in a more beautiful symphony.

3. Warm Up Like A Maestro: Consider your warm-up to be the equivalent of tuning your instrument before a performance. Gentle stretches and gentle activity prepare your muscles and joints to avoid strains and injuries.

4. Buddy Up for Safety: Exercising with a buddy or in a group class increases motivation and social contact, making you more inclined to listen to your body and alter your motions as required.

5. Hydration equals harmony: Stay hydrated before, during, and after your workout to keep your energy levels up and your body lubricated. Dehydration can cause weariness and muscular cramps.

6. Wear the right gear: Uncomfortable clothing and footwear can transform your ecstasy into a dance of irritation. Choose comfortable clothing and shoes with adequate shock absorption. Style and safety may make a beautiful duo!

7. Know Your Limitations: Don't try to run a marathon while your heart is singing the song of a slow waltz. To avoid overexertion and exhaustion, gradually increase both intensity and duration.

8. When the Music Stumbles: Recovery Tips

9. Rest and Repair: If you have an injury, listen to your body and emphasize rest. Allow time for tissues to recover and inflammation to diminish before resuming activity.

10. Seek Medical Advice: If you have a more serious injury, see your doctor or a physiotherapist. They can identify the issue and provide suitable therapy and rehabilitation exercises.

11. Ice the Ache Away: Applying ice packs to the afflicted region might help reduce swelling and discomfort. For best recuperation, use the RICE concept (rest, ice, compression, and elevation).

12. Gentle Movement Is Your Friend While full rest is essential during the early period, mild and painless movements can aid in healing and avoid stiffness. Consult your doctor or physiotherapist about safe workouts.

13. Listen to Your Body's Tempo: Do not hurry your healing! Gradually increase the intensity and duration of your workouts as your discomfort reduces and your strength increases.

14. Fuel Your Recovery: Eating a nutritious diet rich in fruits, vegetables, and whole grains gives your body the resources it requires to recuperate. Stay hydrated and avoid processed meals and sugary beverages.

15. Stay optimistic and active: Recovery can be stressful, but keeping optimistic and active in activities you like will help you feel better and motivate yourself. Consider mild stretching, light gardening, or quality time with loved ones.

Remember, injury prevention and rehabilitation are essential components of your joyful movement symphony. Listening to your body, taking precautions, and prioritizing recovery will allow you to keep the music playing and dance with abandon. So put on your comfy shoes, turn on your favorite music, and enjoy the elegant rhythm of safe and pleasant workout!

Conclusion

Forget the bingo halls and the dusty treadmill. Retirement isn't about waiting for life to happen; it's about becoming the life of the party! Low-impact exercise is more than just a stroll to the checkout line; it's a lively waltz led by laughter. Trade hurting joints for sun-kissed vigor, and replace exhaustion with the euphoria of newly discovered strength.

Every gentle stretch is like a brushstroke on a canvas of vivid health. Each beautiful movement creates a symphony of harmony, confidence, and sheer delight. In the dance floor of life, age is just a number, and you are a seasoned pro ready to take center stage.

So put on your dancing shoes, turn on your favorite music, and take the stage for your own joyous revolution! Leave the pains and limits behind and replace them with salsa grins and tai chi twirls. This isn't a chore; it's a celebration of your wonderful, ageless body, reminding you that you're a dance queen (or king!) yearning to show off your inner groove.

The world is your stage, and the melody of a healthier, happier you is ready to be heard. Take the first step, feel the rhythm running through your veins, and dance your way to a vibrant, joyous existence! Don't wait till tomorrow; take your water bottle, put on your sunshine grin, and begin composing your own movement masterpiece right now! Darling, the curtain is up. **Take a bow, and let the happy symphony of your life begin!**

PROGRESS TRACKER JOURNAL

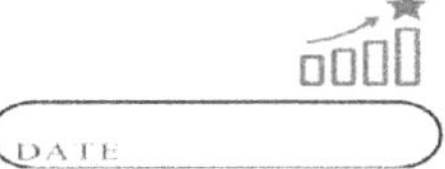

DATE

DAILY AFFIRMATION

WATER TRACKER

EXERCISE LOG

MOOD TRACKER

TODAY I AM GRATEFUL FOR:

1.

2.

3.

MEALS

BREAKFAST

LUNCH

DINNER

SNACKS

DRINKS

THINGS I CAN DO TO MAKE TODAY GREAT:

1.

2.

3.

THREE GREAT THINGS THAT HAPPENED TODAY:

1.

2.

3.

THOUGHTS & REFLECTIONS

PROGRESS TRACKER JOURNAL

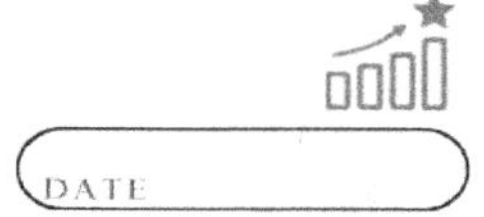

DATE

DAILY AFFIRMATION

WATER TRACKER

EXERCISE LOG

TODAY I AM GRATEFUL FOR:

1.

2.

3.

MOOD TRACKER

MEALS

BREAKFAST

LUNCH

DINNER

SNACKS

DRINKS

THINGS I CAN DO TO MAKE TODAY GREAT:

1.

2.

3.

THREE GREAT THINGS THAT HAPPENED TODAY:

1.

2.

3.

THOUGHTS & REFLECTIONS

PROGRESS TRACKER JOURNAL

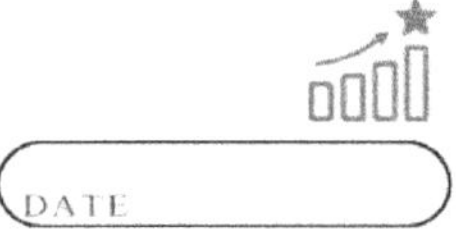

DATE

1.

2.

3.

1.

2.

3.

WATER TRACKER

EXERCISE LOG

MOOD TRACKER

MEALS

BREAKFAST

LUNCH

DINNER

SNACKS

DRINKS

1.

2.

3.

PROGRESS TRACKER JOURNAL

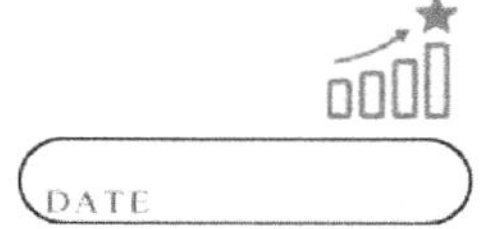

DATE

DAILY AFFIRMATION

WATER TRACKER ○○○○○○○○

EXERCISE LOG

MOOD TRACKER

TODAY I AM GRATEFUL FOR:

MEALS

1.

BREAKFAST

LUNCH

2.

DINNER

SNACKS

3.

DRINKS

THINGS I CAN DO TO MAKE TODAY GREAT:

THREE GREAT THINGS THAT HAPPENED TODAY:

1.

1.

2.

2.

3.

3.

THOUGHTS & REFLECTIONS

PROGRESS TRACKER JOURNAL

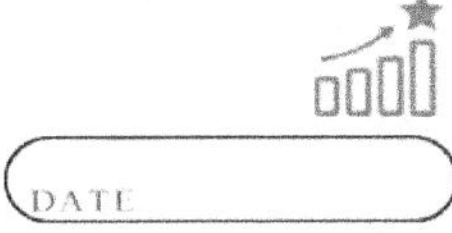

DATE

DAILY AFFIRMATION

WATER TRACKER

EXERCISE LOG

TODAY I AM GRATEFUL FOR:

1.

2.

3.

MOOD TRACKER

MEALS

BREAKFAST

LUNCH

DINNER

SNACKS

DRINKS

THINGS I CAN DO TO MAKE TODAY GREAT:

1.

2.

3.

THREE GREAT THINGS THAT HAPPENED TODAY:

1.

2.

3.

THOUGHTS & REFLECTIONS

PROGRESS TRACKER JOURNAL

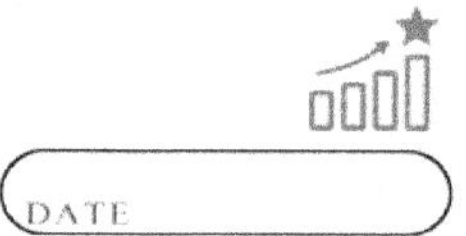

DATE

DAILY AFFIRMATION

WATER TRACKER

EXERCISE LOG

TODAY I AM GRATEFUL FOR:

1.

2.

3.

MOOD TRACKER

MEALS

BREAKFAST

LUNCH

DINNER

SNACKS

DRINKS

THINGS I CAN DO TO MAKE TODAY GREAT:

1.

2.

3.

THREE GREAT THINGS THAT HAPPENED TODAY:

1.

2.

3.

THOUGHTS & REFLECTIONS

PROGRESS TRACKER JOURNAL

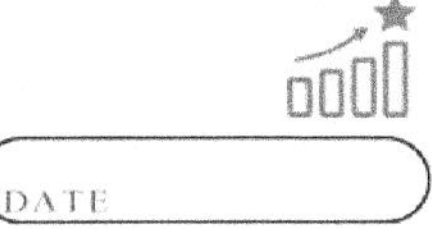

DATE

DAILY AFFIRMATION

TODAY I AM GRATEFUL FOR:

1.

2.

3.

THINGS I CAN DO TO MAKE TODAY GREAT:

1.

2.

3.

THOUGHTS & REFLECTIONS

WATER TRACKER

EXERCISE LOG

MOOD TRACKER

MEALS

BREAKFAST

LUNCH

DINNER

SNACKS

DRINKS

THREE GREAT THINGS THAT HAPPENED TODAY:

1.

2.

3.

PROGRESS TRACKER JOURNAL

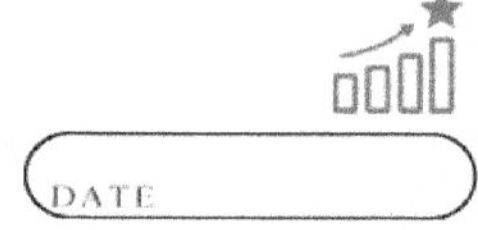

DATE

DAILY AFFIRMATION

TODAY I AM GRATEFUL FOR:

1.

2.

3.

THINGS I CAN DO TO MAKE TODAY GREAT:

1.

2.

3.

THOUGHTS & REFLECTIONS

WATER TRACKER

EXERCISE LOG

MOOD TRACKER

MEALS

BREAKFAST

LUNCH

DINNER

SNACKS

DRINKS

THREE GREAT THINGS THAT HAPPENED TODAY:

1.

2.

3.

PROGRESS TRACKER JOURNAL

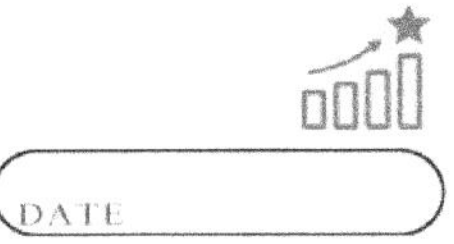

DATE

DAILY AFFIRMATION

WATER TRACKER ○○○○○○○

EXERCISE LOG

MOOD TRACKER ☹ ☹ ☺ ☺ ☺

TODAY I AM GRATEFUL FOR:

MEALS

1.

BREAKFAST

LUNCH

2.

DINNER

SNACKS

3.

DRINKS

THINGS I CAN DO TO MAKE TODAY GREAT:

THREE GREAT THINGS THAT HAPPENED TODAY:

1.

1.

2.

2.

3.

3.

THOUGHTS & REFLECTIONS

PROGRESS TRACKER JOURNAL

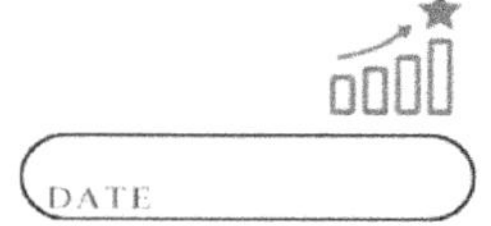

DATE

DAILY AFFIRMATION

WATER TRACKER

EXERCISE LOG

MOOD TRACKER

TODAY I AM GRATEFUL FOR:

1.

2.

3.

MEALS

BREAKFAST

LUNCH

DINNER

SNACKS

DRINKS

THINGS I CAN DO TO MAKE TODAY GREAT:

1.

2.

3.

THREE GREAT THINGS THAT HAPPENED TODAY:

1.

2.

3.

THOUGHTS & REFLECTIONS

PROGRESS TRACKER JOURNAL

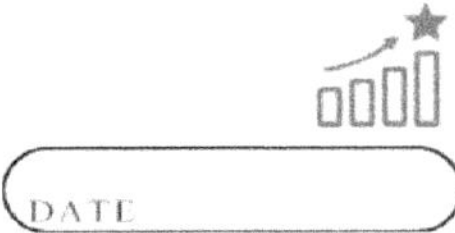

DATE

DAILY AFFIRMATION

TODAY I AM GRATEFUL FOR:

1.

2.

3.

THINGS I CAN DO TO MAKE TODAY GREAT:

1.

2.

3.

THOUGHTS & REFLECTIONS

WATER TRACKER

EXERCISE LOG

MOOD TRACKER

MEALS

BREAKFAST

LUNCH

DINNER

SNACKS

DRINKS

THREE GREAT THINGS THAT HAPPENED TODAY:

1.

2.

3.

PROGRESS TRACKER JOURNAL

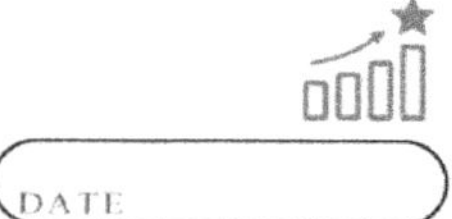

DATE

DAILY AFFIRMATION

WATER TRACKER

EXERCISE LOG

MOOD TRACKER

MEALS

BREAKFAST

LUNCH

DINNER

SNACKS

DRINKS

TODAY I AM GRATEFUL FOR:

1.

2.

3.

THINGS I CAN DO TO MAKE TODAY GREAT:

1.

2.

3.

THREE GREAT THINGS THAT HAPPENED TODAY:

1.

2.

3.

THOUGHTS & REFLECTIONS

PROGRESS TRACKER JOURNAL

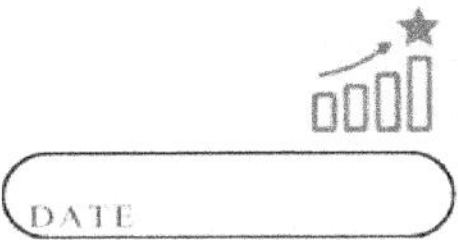

DATE

DAILY AFFIRMATION

TODAY I AM GRATEFUL FOR:

1.

2.

3.

THINGS I CAN DO TO MAKE TODAY GREAT:

1.

2.

3.

THOUGHTS & REFLECTIONS

WATER TRACKER

EXERCISE LOG

MOOD TRACKER

MEALS

BREAKFAST

LUNCH

DINNER

SNACKS

DRINKS

THREE GREAT THINGS THAT HAPPENED TODAY:

1.

2.

3.

PROGRESS TRACKER JOURNAL

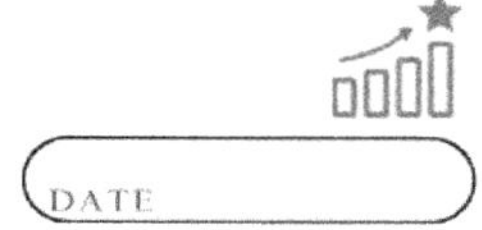

DATE

TODAY I AM GRATEFUL FOR:

1.

2.

3.

THINGS I CAN DO TO MAKE TODAY GREAT:

1.

2.

3.

THOUGHTS & REFLECTIONS

WATER TRACKER

EXERCISE LOG

MOOD TRACKER

MEALS

BREAKFAST

LUNCH

DINNER

SNACKS

DRINKS

THREE GREAT THINGS THAT HAPPENED TODAY:

1.

2.

3.

PROGRESS TRACKER JOURNAL

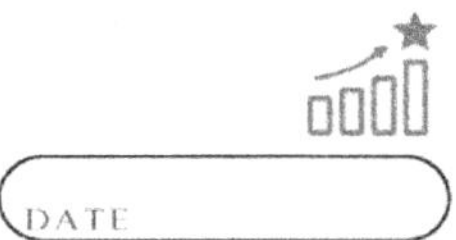

DATE

DAILY AFFIRMATION

WATER TRACKER

EXERCISE LOG

MOOD TRACKER

MEALS

BREAKFAST

LUNCH

DINNER

SNACKS

DRINKS

TODAY I AM GRATEFUL FOR:

1.

2.

3.

THINGS I CAN DO TO MAKE TODAY GREAT:

1.

2.

3.

THREE GREAT THINGS THAT HAPPENED TODAY:

1.

2.

3.

THOUGHTS & REFLECTIONS

PROGRESS TRACKER JOURNAL

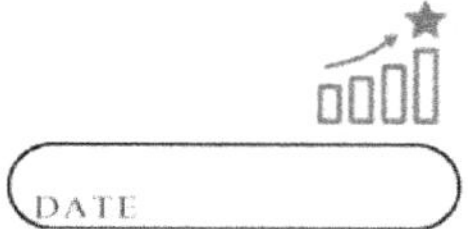

DATE

DAILY AFFIRMATION

WATER TRACKER

EXERCISE LOG

MOOD TRACKER

TODAY I AM GRATEFUL FOR:

1.

2.

3.

MEALS

BREAKFAST

LUNCH

DINNER

SNACKS

DRINKS

THINGS I CAN DO TO MAKE TODAY GREAT:

1.

2.

3.

THREE GREAT THINGS THAT HAPPENED TODAY:

1.

2.

3.

THOUGHTS & REFLECTIONS

PROGRESS TRACKER JOURNAL

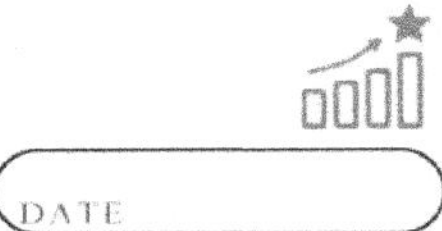

DATE

DAILY AFFIRMATION

TODAY I AM GRATEFUL FOR:

1.

2.

3.

THINGS I CAN DO TO MAKE TODAY GREAT:

1.

2.

3.

THOUGHTS & REFLECTIONS

WATER TRACKER

EXERCISE LOG

MOOD TRACKER

MEALS

BREAKFAST

LUNCH

DINNER

SNACKS

DRINKS

THREE GREAT THINGS THAT HAPPENED TODAY:

1.

2.

3.

PROGRESS TRACKER JOURNAL

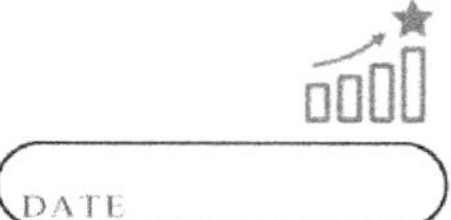

(DATE)

DAILY AFFIRMATION

TODAY I AM GRATEFUL FOR:

1.

2.

3.

THINGS I CAN DO TO MAKE TODAY GREAT:

1.

2.

3.

THOUGHTS & REFLECTIONS

WATER TRACKER

EXERCISE LOG

MOOD TRACKER

MEALS

BREAKFAST

LUNCH

DINNER

SNACKS

DRINKS

THREE GREAT THINGS THAT HAPPENED TODAY:

1.

2.

3.